COMPACT GUIDES TO FITNESS & HEALTH

YOUR HEALTHY BACK

CONTENT PROVIDED BY MAYO CLINIC HEALTH INFORMATION

MASON CREST PUBLISHERS
Philadelphia, Pennsylvania

Your Healthy Back provides reliable, practical, easy-to-understand information on the care of the back and relief from back pain. Much of the information comes directly from the experience of Mayo Clinic physicians, nurses, registered dietitians, health educators and other health care professionals. This book supplements the advice of your personal physician, whom you should consult for individual medical problems. MAYO, MAYO CLINIC, MAYO CLINIC HEALTH INFORMATION and the Mayo triple-shield logo are marks of Mayo Foundation for Medical Education and Research.

Hardcover Library Edition Published 2002
Mason Crest Publishers
370 Reed Road
Suite 302
Broomall, PA 19008-0914
(866) MCP-BOOK (toll free)

First Printing
1 2 3 4 5 6 7 8 9 10
Library of Congress Cataloging-in-Publication Data on file at the Library of Congress

ISBN 1-59084-263-4 (hc)
Printed in the United States of America

Contents

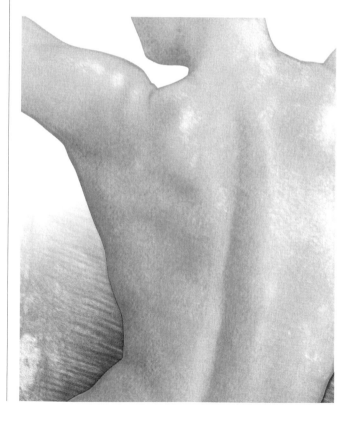

Introduction

You can view back pain simply as a problem to live with — or as a reason to take charge of your health.

If you ever feel back pain, you're not alone. Back pain is one of the most common reasons that people call their doctors.

Yet, you can often prevent back problems with simple steps:

- Take charge of your health with exercise.
- Plan daily activities with your back in mind.
- Learn about sources of back pain.
- Know how to treat back pain yourself — and when to call your doctor.

In addition, learn about common medical treatments for back pain.

Back pain is common, especially as you get older. But it's not inevitable.

What's more, most back pain is short-lived. Up to 90 percent of back pain improves within 6 weeks. Even if you injured your back in the past, you can prevent or reduce pain.

What does your back do?

If you're like most people, you don't think much about your back until it hurts. What does your back actually do for you?

The answer is balance. Cars have four wheels, chairs have four legs, and fellow mammals from mice to monkeys walk on four feet. Four points make balance easy.

But humans balance on two legs — a remarkable feat of engineering. To accomplish this achievement:

- Muscles contract and relax, allowing you to stand and move.
- Tendons fasten muscles to the bones in your back (vertebrae).
- Ligaments (tough, fibrous bands) hold your vertebrae together.
- Your spine protects the spinal cord, the main pathway for your central nervous system.

This intricate network of bones, muscles, ligaments, tendons and nerves (see below) balances and bears the weight of your body, as well as the loads you carry.

Because this network is so complex and so crucial

Your back includes:

- 24 vertebrae
- The sacrum and coccyx (tailbone)
- 31 pairs of nerves
- 40 muscles and many connecting ligaments and tendons running from the base of your skull to your tailbone
- Disks, which are the fibrous, elastic cartilage structures between your vertebrae. Disks act as "shock absorbers" to keep your spine flexible and cushion the hard vertebrae as you move.

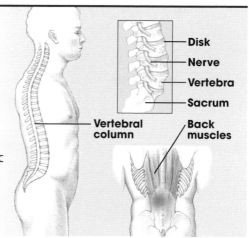

Disk

Nerve

Vertebra

Sacrum

Vertebral column

Back muscles

to daily activities, it's vulnerable to injury, sprain and strain. Minor damage to one part of your back's structure can upset the delicate balance.

Back pain can occur for no apparent reason and at any point on your spine. However, the most common site for pain is your lower back (see below). This area bears the majority of your weight and acts as a pivot point for turning at your waist.

Natural "shock absorber"

Your back has natural curves in your neck, upper back and lower back. This shape helps your back absorb impact. Most complaints of back pain center on the lower back. Because of its frequent and varied motions, your lower back is vulnerable to injury.

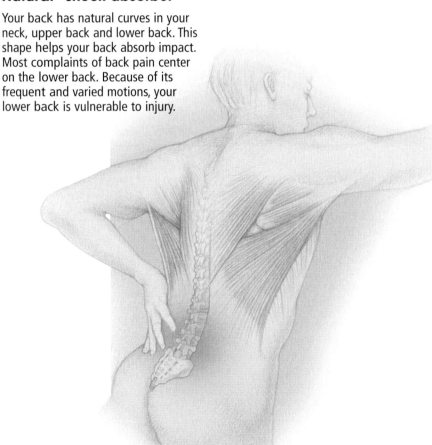

Care for your back with exercise

You can do a lot to protect and preserve the delicate balance in your back. Your most potent tool is regular exercise.

With exercise you can:
- Increase your overall fitness.
- Shed excess pounds that stress your back.
- Stretch and tone your back muscles, and the muscles that support your back, helping you resist injury.
- Reduce your risk of injury by warming up muscles.
- Increase long-term flexibility.

Aerobic exercise gets you breathing harder, delivers more oxygen to your muscles and helps relieve pain. And strength training can decrease your risk of falls and other injuries. Strong arms, legs and abdominal muscles also help relieve back strain. If you have osteoporosis (loss of calcium and weakened bones), back-strengthening exercises can help prevent compression fractures.

"Your daily back routine" on pages 8 to 9 illustrates useful back exercises. If you have osteoporosis, talk to your doctor or a physical therapist before you begin an exercise program.

When you start an exercise program, set a goal of 30 minutes a day for most days of the week. You can do one full session or divide it into two 15-minute sessions or three 10-minute sessions throughout the day. Keep in mind these four general guidelines:

1. Start slowly.
If you're out of condition from lack of activity, your back muscles may be weak and susceptible to injury. When you start exercising, pace yourself. Don't overdo it. Begin gently, and gradually increase your workout time as you become stronger.

2. Choose back-friendly exercise.
When starting an exercise program, choose an activity that is easy on your back:

- *Consider swimming and other water exercises.* Because you don't bear weight during these activities, they place minimal strain on your lower back.
- *Work out on a stationary bike, treadmill or cross-country ski machine.* These forms of exercise jar your back less than running on hard surfaces.
- *Ride a bicycle.* Be sure to adjust the seat and handlebars so that you assume proper posture while pedaling. (For tips on posture, see "Protect your back with careful movement," page 12.)
- *If you play sports, protect your back.* Warm up well and stretch for 10 minutes to prepare for the full range of motion required. (See "Your daily back routine," pages 10 to 11, for stretching exercises.)

3. Avoid high-risk moves.

Activities that involve a lot of twisting, quick stops and sudden starts, and impact on hard surfaces pose the greatest risk to your back. These types of activities include tennis, racquetball, basketball and contact sports such as football.

Also avoid movements that exaggerate the stretch of your muscles. For example, don't try to touch your toes with your legs straight.

4. Reinforce exercise with diet.

Despite the many food fads, no special diet is proven to reverse sources of back pain such as arthritis (inflammation of the joints) or osteoporosis.

However, you can eat a varied diet emphasizing low-fat and high-fiber foods to maintain a healthy weight. Excess pounds add stress to your weight-bearing joints, worsen pain, and promote stiffness and inflammation.

Many people think that choosing a healthy diet requires making drastic changes in what they eat. Often that's not the case at all. A few small, gradual changes can make a big difference in the long run. Follow these tips:

- *Moderate your food intake.* If you eat reasonable portion sizes, it's easier to include all the foods you enjoy and still have a healthy diet.
- *Eat slowly.* It takes about 20 minutes for your brain to receive the signal that you're full. Make sure your meals last at least this long.
- *Try something new.* No single food supplies all the nutrients you need. Increase the variety of foods you eat by trying new fruits and vegetables, whole-grain breads and cereals, and dried peas and beans.
- *Balance your choices over time.* Your food choices over several days should average out to a balance of nutrients. Not every food or meal you eat has to be perfect.
- *Eat three or more calcium-rich foods every day.* These foods help to maintain optimal bone health and prevent age-related bone loss. Calcium-rich foods include milk, yogurt, cheese, canned salmon with bones, collards and calcium-fortified orange juice. Also consume vitamin D to help your body absorb dietary calcium. Ask your doctor or a registered dietitian about ways to get the specific amounts of calcium and vitamin D you need.
- *Limit foods and chemicals that decrease your calcium supply.* A high-protein diet can reduce the amount of calcium your body absorbs. Keep portions of meat, poultry, fish and other protein sources at 5 to 7 ounces daily. Also limit sodium, alcohol and caffeine.

Your daily back routine

Here are basic exercises to stretch and strengthen your back and supporting muscles. Try to work at least 15 minutes of back exercise into your daily routine. Do each exercise three or four times, then increase your goal over time. Remember not to hold your breath. Aerobic exercise aims to help you breathe fully and deeply.

If you have osteoporosis, get medical advice before doing these exercises.

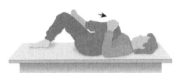

Knee to shoulder stretch — Lie on your back on a firm surface. Bend your knees and keep your feet flat. (This is the starting position.) Pull your left knee toward your chest with both hands. Hold for 15 to 30 seconds. Return to the starting position. Repeat with the opposite leg. Repeat with each leg three or four times.

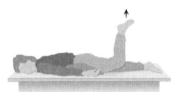

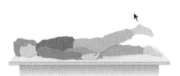

Leg lifts: Step 1 — Lie face down on a firm surface with a large pillow under your hips and lower abdomen. Keeping your knee bent, raise your leg slightly off the surface and hold for about 5 seconds. Repeat several times with both legs.

Leg lifts: Step 2 — Repeat the exercise with your leg straight. Raise one leg slightly off the surface and hold for about 5 seconds. Repeat several times with both legs.

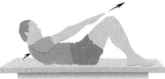

Half sit-up — Lie on your back on a firm surface. Bend your knees and keep your feet flat. (This is the starting position.) Stretch out your arms and reach toward your knees with your hands. Keep reaching until your shoulder blades no longer touch the ground. Do not grasp your knees. Hold for a few seconds and slowly return to the starting position. Repeat several times.

Chair stretch — Sit in a chair. Slowly bend forward toward the floor until you feel a mild stretch in your back. Hold for 15 to 30 seconds. Repeat several times.

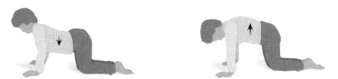

"Cat" stretch — Get down on your hands and knees. Slowly let your back and abdomen sag toward the floor. Slowly arch your back away from the floor. Pull your abdomen up toward the ceiling. Repeat several times.

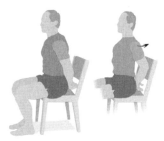

Shoulder blade squeeze — Sit upright in a chair. Keep your chin tucked in and your shoulders down. (This is the starting position.) Pull your shoulder blades together, straighten your upper back, and hold your chest high. Hold for a few seconds. Return to the starting position. Repeat several times.

Protect your back with careful movement

In addition to exercising, you can prevent pain by moving carefully and consciously throughout daily activities. By maintaining your spine's normal curves, you reduce strain on your back. The following ideas can help:

1. Plan your moves.
Reorganize your work and leisure activities to eliminate high-risk, repetitive movements. Avoid unnecessary bending, twisting and reaching. Plan to limit the time you spend carrying heavy briefcases, purses and bags.

2. Listen to your body.
If you must sit or stand for a prolonged period, change your position often. Take at least 30 seconds every 15 minutes to stretch, move or relax. If your back hurts, stop what you're doing and rest.

3. Use the phone wisely.
Avoid holding the telephone with your shoulder while you use your hands to write or do other tasks. If you're on the phone often, use a headset. And as a way to get in the habit of changing positions, stand up whenever you answer the phone.

Posture pointers

A healthy spine (viewed from the side) curves inward at your neck, outward at your upper back, inward at your lower back and outward at your pelvis. Aim to maintain these natural curves.

Standing — Keep your chest held high and your shoulders back and relaxed. Hold in your stomach and buttock muscles. Keep your knees straight (not locked) and your feet parallel.

Sitting — Rest your feet flat on the floor with knees at the same level as your hips.

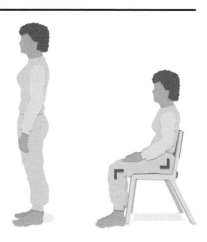

Proper sleeping positions

Avoid aggravating your back when you sleep or lie down:

- Sleep on your stomach only if a pillow cushions your abdomen.
- If you sleep on your back, support your knees and neck with pillows.
- Best option: Sleep on your side with your thighs drawn up somewhat toward your chest. Place a pillow between your legs.

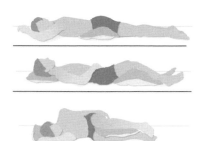

4. Stand smart.

Poor posture stresses your back. When you slouch or stand with a swayback, you exaggerate your back's natural curves. Any imbalance can stress muscles and joints, causing fatigue and injury from overuse. In contrast, good posture relaxes your muscles and uses minimal effort to balance your body.

It's easy to forget these points in the midst of a hectic day. Start by observing your standing position. If you stand for long periods of time, rest one foot on a stool or small box from time to time. While you stand, hold reading material at eye level. And don't bend forward to do desk work or hand work.

5. Sit smart.

Sitting can stress your back. To promote comfort and good posture:

- Choose a chair that supports your lower back.
- Adjust your chair so that your feet stay flat on the floor.
- Place a rolled towel in the small of your back when you sit or drive.
- When you drive, adjust your seat to keep your thighs level. Move your seat forward to avoid overreaching for the pedals.
- Remove a large wallet or any other bulky objects from your back pockets when you sit because they disrupt balance in your lower back.

6. Sleep smart.

Lie on a firm mattress. Use pillows for support, but don't use a pillow that forces your neck up at a severe angle.

7. Plan before you lift.

Before you lift a load, decide where you'll place it and how to get it there. Remember that pushing is safer than pulling. Place heavy objects on casters.

Always bend your knees so that your arms are level with the object you want to lift. Avoid lifting objects over your head. Use a footstool to reach high objects.

8. Prevent falls.

Falls can seriously injure your back, especially if you have osteoporosis. In older adults, falls often lead to broken bones and related back problems.

To prevent falls:
- Wear low-heeled shoes with nonslip soles.
- Walk regularly to maintain coordination and balance.
- Exercise in water.
- Organize your living space to prevent falls. (See "Make your home fall-proof," page 15.)
- See your doctor if you've fallen recently or believe you're at increased risk of falling.

Lift properly

- Plant your feet firmly. Point your toes slightly outward and put one foot slightly ahead of the other. Stand as close to the load as possible.

- Bend from your knees. Use your leg muscles to lift the load. Keep your back as upright as possible. As you lift, tighten the abdominal muscles that support your spine. Check the weight of the load.

- Hold the load close to your body. Avoid turning or twisting while holding the load. Avoid lifting heavy loads above your waist.

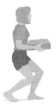

Make your home fall-proof

Your home can literally trip you up. However, you can prevent falls with simple corrective actions:

- Keep electrical and telephone cords tucked out of the way.
- Arrange furniture so that you can move around it easily.
- Get rid of throw rugs, and make sure carpeting is secured to the floor.
- Make sure you can rise from chairs and couches without straining your back.
- Use a stepstool when you need something from a high shelf. Move often-used items to a lower shelf.
- Install grab bars on walls around the tub and beside the toilet.
- Use nonskid mats, adhesive strips or carpet on surfaces that may get wet.
- Place light switches within reach of your bed.
- Install a night light between the bedroom and bathroom.
- Make sure you can reach the telephone from your bed. When you do get up from bed, do so slowly to avoid dizziness, which may cause you to fall.
- Buy nightwear that's short enough so that you won't trip over it.
- Keep stairways, hallways and pathways free of clutter. Check to see that these areas are well lit.
- Install handrails on both sides of stairs.
- Apply brightly colored tape to the face of the steps to make them more visible.
- Purchase a cordless phone to carry with you so you don't have to hurry to answer the phone.
- If you're worried that you may not be able to get up from a fall, consider a personal emergency response system. Pressing a button on this device sends an alert to your clinic. Ask your doctor about this option.

Balance yourself with tai chi

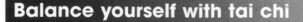

One sophisticated and enjoyable method to improve balance is an ancient form of exercise called tai chi (TIE-chee). Originally developed in China, tai chi involves slow, gentle, dance-like movements that relax and strengthen muscles and joints.

Research indicates that tai chi can prevent falls in older adults by improving strength and balance. In one large study, those who practiced tai chi reduced their risk of falls by about 47 percent.

You'll find tai chi classes offered in cities throughout the United States. To locate a class in your community, contact your local senior center, YMCA or health club.

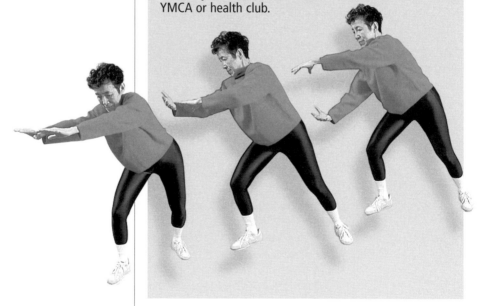

Use corsets with caution

You can buy back braces and corsets over-the-counter or by prescription for about $35. Most full-service pharmacies and medical supply stores stock them.

Worn properly, braces and corsets relieve strain. They can also provide warmth, comfort and support to your back.

Unfortunately, braces and corsets that provide adequate support may also have stiff stays and uncomfortable shoulder straps. Another drawback: Because support comes from the corset rather than your own muscles, a corset may actually weaken your back muscles. This can happen if you wear corsets for long periods of time.

Most experts recommend using braces and corsets for short periods or only during back-straining activities.

At work, some people wear a lightweight, wide elastic or Lycra mesh belt around the lower back and across the abdomen. These specially designed supports compress the abdomen and provide additional support to the spine. To use them effectively:

- Wear the belt only when you have to lift — not for your whole shift.

- Adjust the belt so that the top is at your belly button. The biggest mistake people make is to wear the belts at their waist, over their midsection and too high. Tip: Move it down.

- Adjust the suspenders over your shoulders, but remember they are there only to keep the belt in place if you unfasten it.

- Attend a back safety program to learn how to lift. Don't attempt to lift or move anything heavier than you might without the belt.

- When the Velcro wears out or the mesh tears, get a new belt. Lycra mesh belts may last several months with daily use.

Prevent common sources of back pain

To stay in charge of your health, prevent common sources of back pain. (See "Common sources of back pain," page 20.)

In many cases, you can manage back problems long before they turn into conditions that call for medical treatment. This booklet explains several important prevention strategies in detail, including:
- Exercise (page 7)
- Good posture (page 12)
- Smart lifting (page 14)
- Ways to prevent falls (page 15)

Also keep these three ideas in mind:

1. Reduce stress.

Stress produces physical symptoms including back pain, headaches, constipation, high blood pressure, insomnia, frequent illness and more. On a psychological level, stress can surface in many ways. Examples are anxiety, sadness, irritability, racing thoughts and feelings of hopelessness.

To prevent these symptoms, learn to reduce stress. Begin with these strategies:
- *Relax.* Techniques such as guided imagery, meditation, muscle relaxation and deep breathing can help you relax. So can regular massage. (See "Massage: The lowdown on rubdowns," page 29.)
- *Seek emotional support.* When you feel stressed, talk with a trusted friend. Doing so helps you gain perspective and plan effective action.
- *Simplify your life.* Focus on the people and projects most important to you. Say no to lower-priority commitments that will send your schedule into overdrive.
- *Break large tasks down into smaller steps.* Then focus your attention on accomplishing the small steps, one at a time.

2. Sleep well.

We live in a sleep-deprived culture. Some people even boast about how little they sleep. However, back pain makes it essential for you to get enough rest. Sleep as many hours as you need, not as many as you think you should. Consider taking 20- to 30-minute naps during the afternoon. But avoid naps if they interfere with night sleep.

3. Schedule regular medical exams.

In general, you should get a complete physical twice in your 20s, three times in your 30s, four times in your 40s, five times in your 50s, and annually after that. If you feel back pain — especially when it lasts more than 6 weeks — be sure to tell your doctor.

Doctors can detect some sources of back pain and treat them in early stages. Sometimes new technology makes this possible. For example, bone sonometers assess the risk for osteoporosis in about 1 minute. These devices use high-frequency sound waves to measure bone density in the foot.

Common sources of back pain

• **Degenerative disk disease**. With age, your disks become worn and the spaces between your vertebrae narrow. This is called degenerative disk disease, but it's really part of the normal aging process. About 1 in 100 people will also develop a nerve irritation, signaled by aches and pains in the leg and back. For example, people with back pain often talk about "slipped disks." Actually, disks don't slip. But they can bulge or rupture (herniate). When this happens, parts of the disk protrude from their normal position between your vertebrae. Pain can result when a fragment of the herniated disk places pressure on an adjacent nerve. (See "Sciatica" below.)

• **Osteoarthritis**. This condition affects cartilage, a rubbery tissue that covers the ends of your bones and lies between weight-bearing joints. Cartilage is normally smooth so that your joints can move easily but remain firm and supple to absorb shock. As osteoarthritis progresses, surfaces of cartilage and underlying bone become compressed and irregular. Bony outgrowths called spurs may form. Instead of gliding smoothly, joint surfaces rub against each other.

• **Sciatica (sy-AT-i-kuh)**. This condition gets its name from the sciatic nerve that extends down each leg from your buttock to your heel. Sciatica happens when nerves in your lower back or buttocks are inflamed or compressed. You feel pain from your back down through your lower leg. Tingling, numbness or muscle weakness may also accompany nerve compression. The pain from sciatica usually resolves on its own, but it's good to get a doctor's evaluation.

• **Osteoporosis**. This term literally means "porous bones." Osteoporosis happens when loss of calcium weakens your bone structure. The amount of calcium in your bones decreases as you age. Bones that were once strong can become weak and brittle — so brittle that even mild stresses like bending to pick up a newspaper, lifting a vacuum, coughing or a strong hug can cause a fracture. In some cases, the vertebrae become compressed, resulting in back pain. Progressive compression of vertebrae often leads to a gradual loss of height, especially in women after menopause.

• **Fibromyalgia (fy-bro-my-AL-juh)**. This disorder is often called fibromyalgia syndrome, referring not to a specific illness but to a condition that involves many symptoms. The main symptom of fibromyalgia is chronic pain — "aching all over." You may feel the pain as a deep ache or burning sensation. You may also experience stiffness and discomfort in your muscles, tendons and ligaments. However, having fibromyalgia does not mean that your joints are inflamed or damaged.

Treat back pain with self-care

The vast majority of back problems are not disabling or life-threatening. The first line of treatment for back pain is self-care that you can do at home.

Seventy percent of people with back pain find that their pain improves in 2 to 3 weeks with simple measures like rest and over-the-counter pain relievers. If you have disk-related pain, your recovery could take longer. But with time and proper care, you can overcome even pain from a herniated disk.

Begin your program of self-care with the following treatments:

Apply cold, then heat

To soothe sore, inflamed muscles, use sources of heat and cold, including hot baths and hot or cold compresses.

For the first 2 days after an injury, use cold treatment:

1. Put ice in a plastic bag. You can also use an ice pack or bag of frozen vegetables.
2. Wrap the bag or pack in a cloth or towel. Keeping a thin barrier between the ice and your skin prevents frostbite.
3. Hold the bag or pack on the sore area four times a day. You can do this for up to 15 minutes at a time. Do not go longer than 15 minutes.

Use this cold treatment for as long as spasms persist — usually 48 hours. After that you can apply heat to help further loosen tight muscles:

- Use a heating pad, heat lamp, warm compress or warm bath.
- Limit each heat application to 20 minutes.
- To avoid burns, keep heating pads on a low setting and away from areas of reduced sensation.

Even after you start heat treatment, you might find that cold gives you more relief. In that case, continue using cold treatment. Or combine cold and hot treatments.

Tests help with diagnosis

The causes of back pain are many, and pinpointing the source may take time. In some cases, you may never know the cause. In seeking a diagnosis, your doctor may use some of the following tests:

X-rays
These tests can reveal vertebrae problems, tumors or degenerative changes in your spine. Yet, a growing consensus of experts suggests that X-rays are generally not needed for most acute cases of lower back pain.

Computed tomography (CT)
Using computers and X-rays, CT scanners form a series of cross-sectional images that can define disk and other problems.

Myelography
Myelography (my-eh-LOG-ruh-fee) involves a special dye that's injected into your spinal canal. After the injection, X-rays of your vertebrae can reveal a herniated disk or other lesions.

Magnetic resonance imaging (MRI)
An MRI machine combines a strong magnetic force with radio waves. The result: computer-generated images of bones, muscles, cartilage, ligaments, tendons and blood vessels. MRI testing can identify herniated disks or other problems with your back.

Electrodiagnostic studies
These tests measure the electrical impulses produced by the nerves in your muscles. Studies of your nerve pathways can confirm nerve compression caused by herniated disks or spinal stenosis.

Bone scans
During a bone scan, a radiologist injects a radioactive substance (tracer) into one of your veins. Doctors then use a special camera to locate bone tumors or compression fractures caused by osteoporosis.

Understand your treatment options

Persistent back pain calls for professional treatment, which can include any of the options below. Even if you receive such treatments, your doctor will probably recommend that you continue regular self-care and exercise. (See "Care for your back with exercise," page 7.) Tell your primary doctor about all treatments — both traditional and alternative — that you receive for back pain.

Education and "back schools"
You can play a major role in managing and preventing back pain. Learn all you can about how to protect your back, the role of exercise, and your options for treatment. Ask your doctor for reading materials. Ask questions if you have concerns or don't understand your doctor's recommendations.

Many communities offer "back schools" — classes that can teach you ways to manage and prevent back pain. Classroom study generally focuses on back anatomy and function. That's followed by practice sessions with exercises that help you protect your back at home and work. To enter back school, you may need a doctor's referral.

Prescription medications
Typical medications include over-the-counter pain relievers, such as acetaminophen, and nonsteroidal anti-inflammatory drugs (NSAIDs), such as ibuprofen. Some drugs, like muscle relaxants, are available only with a prescription.

For pain relief, your doctor may prescribe both a muscle relaxant and an NSAID. These are usually short-term medications.

Epidural steroid injections
Epidural steroid injections may be recommended when pain doesn't respond to simpler measures. These injections may help relieve inflammation in the epidural space that surrounds your spinal cord.

It involves using a needle to inject cortisone (an anti-inflammatory) into the epidural space to decrease inflammation and swelling of the nerves, reducing pain and other symptoms.

This procedure is done on an outpatient basis using a local anesthetic to numb the skin and surrounding tissues. If the first injection doesn't reduce pain after about 2 weeks, a second and possibly a third injection might be recommended. Epidural injections may reduce back pain for some people, but not everyone.

Physical therapy and rehabilitation

Your primary care doctor may refer you to a doctor (physiatrist) who specializes in physical medicine and rehabilitation (PM&R). These doctors focus on restoring function, treating low back pain and many other musculoskeletal problems. The physiatrist may offer a number of treatment options, based on your diagnosis and whether the pain is acute or chronic.

Once acute pain improves, or if you have chronic symptoms, your doctor or a physical therapist may design a rehabilitation program for you. Physical therapy may include applications of heat or cold or gentle massage that may relieve back pain due to muscle spasms.

Rehabilitation typically involves exercises to help correct your posture, strengthen your back and abdominal muscles, and improve your flexibility. (See "Your daily back routine," pages 10 to 11.) It may also include aerobic conditioning.

Your doctor or physical therapist may offer you the option of electrical stimulation as part of your pain management plan (see below).

Electrical stimulation: TENS and PENS

TENS stands for transcutaneous electrical nerve stimulation. This treatment is intended to prevent pain signals from reaching your brain.

Small electrodes contained in pads are taped to your skin, near the area of pain. The electrodes are attached to a small stimulator, which delivers a tiny electrical current to key points on nerve pathways. The current isn't painful. TENS is thought to work by stimulating the release of endorphins.

TENS works best when used for acute pain associated with a pinched nerve, such as sciatica. It's less successful for chronic pain.

Percutaneous electrical nerve stimulation (PENS) also uses electrical signals to prevent pain messages from traveling to your brain. This treatment involves thin, needle-like electrodes that are inserted into the soft tissues or muscles in your back.

Chiropractic care

A 1992 policy statement from the American Medical Association permits physicians to work with chiropractors — if physicians believe that chiropractic treatment offers a clear benefit. Though they can't prescribe drugs or perform surgery, chiropractors use many standard medical procedures.

Most chiropractors use a hands-on type of adjustment called spinal manipulation. Spinal manipulation can effectively treat *uncomplicated* back pain, especially if the pain has been present for less than 4 weeks.

People other than chiropractors do spinal manipulation. Many osteopathic doctors and physical therapists are trained in this treatment. And there is no evidence that chiropractors do better spinal manipulation than other health care providers.

If you're thinking of seeing a chiropractor, keep the following points in mind:
- First, see the physician who provides your primary medical treatment. If you want spinal manipulation, ask your physician if it's appropriate. Manipulation of your spine can aggravate a disk problem or cause compression fractures if you have osteoporosis.

- If you seek chiropractic care without a referral, do so carefully. Find someone who attended a school accredited by the Council on Chiropractic Education.
- See only chiropractors who are willing to report to your physician, review recent X-ray films provided by your physician, give you a written treatment plan and allow your physician to observe chiropractic treatments.
- Avoid chiropractors who view spinal manipulation as a treatment or cure for a wide range of diseases. There is no evidence to support this idea.

Medicare, Medicaid, health maintenance organizations (HMOs) and other insurers may provide some reimbursement for the services of chiropractors. However, coverage may be limited; check with your insurer.

Acupuncture

An acupuncturist inserts hair-thin needles under your skin, causing little or no pain. The needles usually stay in for 15 to 30 minutes and several sessions may be needed. Research suggests pain relief may come from the release of endorphins, your body's natural painkillers.

Although noting a lack of rigorously controlled research about the benefits of acupuncture, in 1998 the National Institutes of Health (NIH) released a consensus statement saying that acupuncture may help conditions that involve chronic pain, including low back pain.

Pain specialists at Mayo Clinic have used acupuncture since 1974 as one part of a comprehensive treatment program, along with traditional methods such as medication or surgery.

To find a qualified practitioner, ask for a referral from your physician or contact the American Academy of Medical Acupuncture (AAMA). Visit

Massage: The lowdown on rubdowns

For decades the mere mention of massage evoked images of the seedy side of town. No longer. Today, massage is an integral part of physical therapy, sports medicine and nursing care. It's also becoming more accepted as a simple means for healthy people to relieve emotional stress and just feel good.

Massage is the kneading, stroking and manipulation of the soft tissues of your body — your skin, muscles, tendons and ligaments. Your massage will vary depending on the rhythm, rate, pressure and direction of these movements.

A good massage helps you both physically and psychologically. Massage can relax your muscles, increase circulation, reduce swelling and relieve pain. This treatment can also soften scars and decrease adhesions (fibrous tissue that causes other tissue to adhere abnormally).

Massage isn't the answer to all health problems. In fact, some people shouldn't get a massage. For example, you shouldn't have massage over an open wound, skin infection, phlebitis or areas of weakened bones. Also, if you've been injured, consult your doctor. Don't rely exclusively on massage to repair damaged tissues.

Generally, a massage should feel good. If it doesn't, speak up promptly.

When selecting a massage therapist, examine the person's credentials. If your state doesn't require licensing, contact the American Massage Therapy Association at 847-864-0123 or visit its Web site at *www.amtamassage.org*.

the AAMA Web site at *www.medicalacupuncture.org* or call 323-937-5514. AAMA's members are all licensed physicians with more than 200 hours of special training in acupuncture.

Surgery
Odds are you probably won't need surgery for your back pain. Even the pain and disability caused by a herniated disk or spinal stenosis (narrowing of your spinal canal) often decrease with more conservative treatments. Surgery is usually reserved for times when a severely pinched nerve threatens to cause permanent muscle weakness, or when back problems affect bowel or bladder control.

Before you agree to back surgery, consider getting a second opinion. Surgery to remove a herniated disk (laminectomy) or fuse vertebrae (fusion) in the lower back are frequently performed procedures in the United States. (See "Surgery may relieve pressure, add stability," page 31.) However, the long-term outcome for your back may be the same whether you have surgery or choose a less invasive treatment.

Vertebroplasty
Today, less invasive techniques such as vertebroplasty (ver-TEE-bro-plasty) are becoming more common. This involves injecting bone cement into fractured and collapsed vertebrae. The cement hardens over a few hours, sealing and stabilizing fractures and relieving pain. If you have prolonged, severe pain from a compression fracture, you might be a candidate, though some still consider this an experimental treatment.

Surgery may relieve pressure, add stability

Three basic types of back surgery include:

Laminectomy

Laminectomy (lam-ih-NEK-tuh-me) relieves leg pain by removing bone spurs or disk fragments that protrude into your spinal canal or press on nerve roots within your spine. The primary purpose of this procedure is to preserve nerve and muscle function rather than to simply relieve pain.

Diskectomy

This procedure involves the removal of a portion of a disk to relieve pressure on a nerve.

Fusion

Spinal fusion permanently connects two or more bones in your spine to improve stability, correct a deformity or treat pain. To fuse the spine, small pieces of extra bone are needed to fill the space between two vertebrae (the disk is removed first if the front of the spine is fused).

This bone may come from your own body (usually your pelvic bone) or a bone bank. Sometimes wires, rods, screws, metal cages or plates are also used, especially if the spine is unstable or the operation is needed to correct a deformity.

Fusion has a drawback: Decreasing the motion at one point in the spine transfers stress to other points. This can have detrimental effects on the unfused vertebrae.

In the future, other surgeries may help to relieve pain without restricting motion.

Remember back care basics

Take stock of your back and how you use it. You can avoid many back problems by using the main ideas in this booklet:

- Maintain a program of regular, back-friendly exercise (see page 7).
- During everyday activities, use your back muscles with care (see page 12).
- If you have back pain, start with self-care — rest, medication and hot or cold treatments at home (see page 21).
- Call your doctor when self-care doesn't stop the pain within 72 hours. Call immediately if the pain could signal another medical problem (see page 22).

Some people feel helpless about back pain and resign themselves to discomfort. In almost all cases, that attitude is unnecessary.

Empower yourself. Knowledge combined with sensible habits can keep you and your back strong, healthy partners for a lifetime.

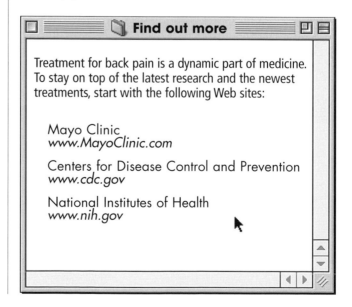

📖 **Find out more**

Treatment for back pain is a dynamic part of medicine. To stay on top of the latest research and the newest treatments, start with the following Web sites:

Mayo Clinic
www.MayoClinic.com

Centers for Disease Control and Prevention
www.cdc.gov

National Institutes of Health
www.nih.gov

GLOSSARY

Bone sonometer: A device used to assess the risk of osteoporosis by using high-frequency sound waves to measure bone density in the foot.

Coccyx: The end of the vertebral column, also known as the tailbone.

Osteoporosis: A bone-weakening disease caused by a gradual loss of calcium and other minerals from bones, making them thinner, weaker and prone to fracture.

Percutaneous electrical nerve stimulation (PENS): Treatment intended to prevent pain signals from reaching your brain through the use of an electrical current. Needle-like electrodes are inserted into soft tissues or muscles in your back.

Physiatrist: A doctor who specializes in physical medicine and rehabilitation. This doctor focuses on restoring function, treating low back pain and other musculoskeletal problems.

Sacrum: The part of the vertebral column that connects to the pelvis.

Tai chi: An ancient form of exercise, developed in China. It involves slow, gentle, dance-like movements that relax and strengthen muscles and joints.

Transcutaneous electrical nerve stimulation (TENS): Treatment intended to prevent pain signals from reaching your brain through the use of an electrical current. Electrodes are placed on the skin near the area of pain.

INDEX